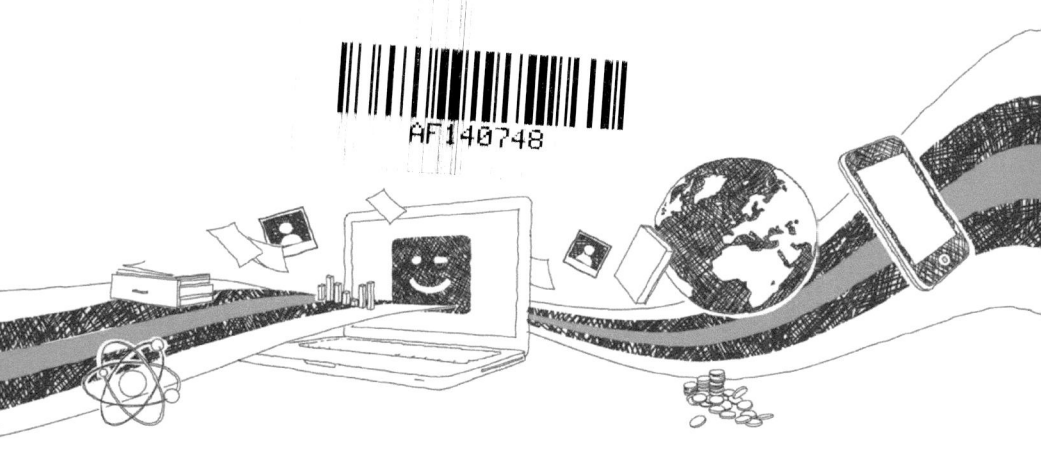
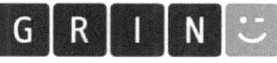

Bibliographic information published by the German National Library:

The German National Library lists this publication in the National Bibliography; detailed bibliographic data are available on the Internet at http://dnb.dnb.de .

Imprint:

Copyright © 2019 GRIN Verlag
Print and binding: Books on Demand GmbH, Norderstedt Germany
ISBN: 9783668963870

This book at GRIN:

https://www.grin.com/document/491644

Julius Holaus

Artificial intelligence in healthcare. An analysis of the link of AI to health promotion and prevention programs to face and early-detect non-communicable diseases

GRIN Verlag

GRIN - Your knowledge has value

Since its foundation in 1998, GRIN has specialized in publishing academic texts by students, college teachers and other academics as e-book and printed book. The website www.grin.com is an ideal platform for presenting term papers, final papers, scientific essays, dissertations and specialist books.

Visit us on the internet:

http://www.grin.com/

http://www.facebook.com/grincom

http://www.twitter.com/grin_com

Artificial intelligence in healthcare – an analysis of the link of AI to health promotion and prevention programs to face and early-detect non-communicable diseases.

LITERATURE REVIEW

Master Program:
"International Business and Law"
Management Center Innsbruck

Lecture:
Academic & Business Writing

Author:
Julius Holaus

ABSTRACT

The global challenge against non-communicable diseases gained transnational attention over the last years. Statistics illustrate, that approximately 70% of all deaths worldwide can be traced back to chronic diseases (WHO, 2014). On the other hand, artificial intelligence is on the rise as the number of implemented software featuring machine-learning skills increased tremendously in the last years. Therefore, the purpose of this literature review is to combine those aspects in order to create synergies of the link between existing approaches with the aim to face non-communicable diseases and artificial intelligence. The review focusses firstly specifically only on the most prevalent NCDs and their characteristics before analysing the rise of machine-learning software from the very beginning. In a next step, those two fields will be combined with the aim to point out both benefits and risks when implementing AI in the healthcare sector. The outcome was, that the use of such software would definitely cut a three-digit number of billions of Euros of spending on healthcare due to the possibility to early-detect diseases and the hereby arising possibility to treat patients in a more efficient way as until now. On the other hand, the biggest risk will be, that artificial intelligence works on huge datasets that need to be set up first – during the setting up process of such data, failures can take place which would have a grave impact on further use.

TABLE OF CONTENTS

LIST OF FIGURES

1. INTRODUCTION

Non-communicable diseases (hereinafter referred to as NCDs) are omnipresent, 95% of the world's population are suffering from at least one burden, every third person suffers from more than five physical deficiencies (Neue Züricher Zeitung, 2015). Chronic diseases cause nearly 40 million deaths per year, which is equivalent to 70% of all deaths globally. The four major and most prevalent NCDs are cardiovascular diseases, cancer, chronic respiratory diseases and diabetes – these physical deficiencies account for most NCD global deaths (WHO, 2014). In Europe, these four NCDs "account for nearly 86% of deaths and 77% of disease burden" (WHO Regional Office for Europe, N.D.) while the population in developing countries seems to be the most vulnerable group of people, as 85% of the ~14 Million deaths caused by NCDs between the ages 30 and 70 are noticed in developing countries (WHO, 2014). Behaviour factors such as tobacco use, excessive alcohol consumption, physical inactivity and unhealthy eating habits increase the risk of dying from NCDs significantly. Furthermore, rapid unplanned urbanization, globalization and population aging are forces, that are responsible for the rising prevalence of chronic diseases over the past years (WHO, 2017).

To break these numbers down into the population of Tyrol, the health report published in 2013 by the Tyrolean provincial government was analysed. According to the *Tiroler Gesundheitsbericht 2012* (Amt der Tiroler Landesregierung, 2013), from 2006 – 2011 an annual death rate of slightly more than 2.700 women was observed. From these 2.740 annual deaths:

~ 1.250 were caused by cardiovascular diseases

~ 660 were caused by cancer

~ 150 were caused by chronic respiratory diseases

From 2006 – 2011 an annual average death rate of 2.510 men was noticed. From these 2.510 annual deaths:

~ 870 were caused by cardiovascular diseases

~ 760 were caused by cancer

~ 190 were caused by chronic respiratory diseases

An analysis of the disease pattern in Tyrol showed, that cardiovascular diseases, cancer and chronic respiratory diseases are the main causes of deaths in that region.

Nevertheless, NCDs do not only affect the health condition and therefore the living standard of people – the WHO Regional Office for Europe (WHO Regional Office for Europe, N.D.) stated in a factsheet, that socioeconomic consequences such as poverty are closely linked with chronic diseases as the healthcare costs for them can quickly drain the household resources of patients. Moreover, vulnerable and socially disadvantaged people get sicker and die sooner due to a greater risk of being exposed to harmful products such as tobacco or alcohol and limited access to health services. Furthermore, a connection between NCDs and economic productivity can be noticed. When taking a closer look at this connection it has been estimated, that "*for every 10% increase in NCD mortality, economic growth is reduced by 0.5%*" (WHO Regional Office for Europe, N.D.). Besides that, the disability, which emerges from being affected by a chronic disease "*can lead to a decrease in working-age population participation in the labour force and reduce productivity and, in turn, reduce per capita gross domestic product growth*" (Engelgau, Rosenhouse, et al., 2011)

All this information leads up to the question on how we can use modern resources like artificial intelligence in a variety of processes within the healthcare sector in order to firstly decrease the possibility to suffer from one of the abovementioned diseases and secondly to treat patients in the most efficient way possible. To analyse the status quo this literature review is structured as follows: first of all, a rough overview of the term "non-communicable diseases" will be given whilst explaining the clinical picture of the most prevalent ones. Afterwards, two common approaches on how to face chronic diseases will be discussed before leading over to the term "artificial intelligence". In the first place, this term will be defined, followed up by the historical development of this specific field in order to gather a broader understanding about its functioning. Lastly, the link between artificial intelligence and the healthcare sector will be outlined – benefits and risks of an implementation will be discussed in order to provide the reader with some objective information.

2. NON-COMMUNICABLE DISEASES

In the following chapters the term non-communicable diseases (NCDs) and its different characteristics will be explained. Burdens which are caused by chronic diseases will be outlined and challenges that occur when facing NCDs will be analysed.

After a brief definition by the WHO, the focus will then be drawn especially on cardiovascular diseases, cancer and diabetes, as those burdens are the most prevalent ones worldwide but also in Tyrol. Additionally, most people who die from NCDs die from those diseases, therefore the necessity to take a closer look at this problem is definitively given.

Furthermore, the difference between health promotion programs and prevention programs will be outlined – the focus will be drawn especially to primary, secondary and tertiary prevention but also to different prevention approaches.

2.1 GENERAL INFORMATION ABOUT THE MOST PREVALENT NCDs

The characteristics of NCDs are, that they are "*a result of a combination of genetic, physiological, environmental and behaviours factors*" (WHO, 2017) – furthermore, they tend to be of long duration and slow progression.

The main NCDs, the ones whose prevalence and death rate is the highest, are cardiovascular diseases, different variations of cancer and diabetes. In the following section, CVDs, cancer and diabetes will be explained briefly in order to get a rough overview on what those diseases are about.

Cardiovascular Diseases

The term "cardiovascular diseases" is used as an umbrella phrase for a variety of diseases of both the heart and blood vessels. The main trigger for CVDs is arteriosclerosis, which describes the ageing process of the blood vessels and therefore their loss of elasticity or their narrowing. Usually, the symptoms of arteriosclerosis remain undiscovered until the vessel diameter is reduced significantly. Nevertheless, the progress of arteriosclerosis is determined by several physical, environmental, social and behaviours factors. (Griebler, Anzenberger & Eisenmann, 2014)

Cancer

Cancer is a disease, that can arise in many different variations: lung cancer, breast cancer, bowel cancer – just to name a few. Also, cancer is not one single disease, "*it is actually a group of more than a hundred diseases that have one basic thing in common: A change occurs in the body that causes cells to grow and multiply uncontrollably*" (Silverstein, A., Silverstein, L., & Silverstein, V., 2006).

The World Cancer Report (International Agency for Research on Cancer, 2014), which was published in 2014 by the International Agency for Research on Cancer, a department administered by the WHO, gave detailed information on both the current situation with cancer and future perspectives but also focused on prevention programmes. According to the report, in 2012 approximately 14 million new cases of cancer and about 8 million cancer-related deaths were observed. The most prevalent sites of cancer can be found in *Figure 1*.

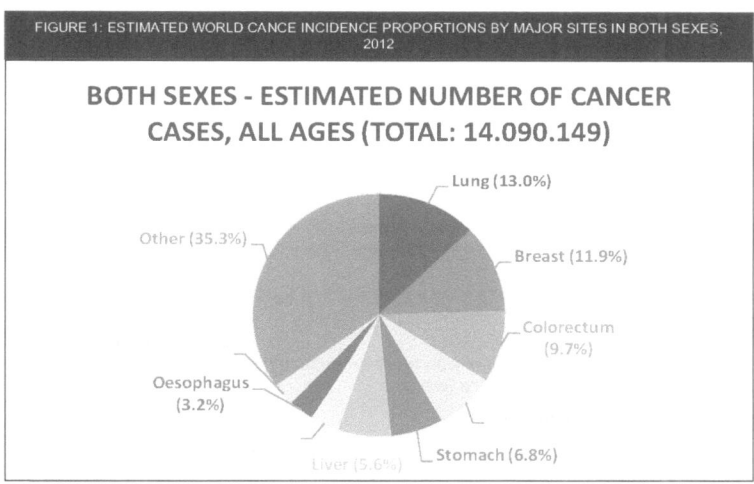

FIGURE 1: ESTIMATED WORLD CANCE INCIDENCE PROPORTIONS BY MAJOR SITES IN BOTH SEXES, 2012

BOTH SEXES - ESTIMATED NUMBER OF CANCER CASES, ALL AGES (TOTAL: 14.090.149)

Lung (13.0%)
Other (35.3%)
Breast (11.9%)
Colorectum (9.7%)
Oesophagus (3.2%)
Liver (5.6%)
Stomach (6.8%)

(based on: International Agency for Research on Cancer, 2014)

Diabetes (Mellitus)

Diabetes mellitus– commonly used as Diabetes – is basically a metabolic disorder, which leads to a high blood sugar level. The level can increase until the sugar gets exuded with urine, because the kidneys cannot hold back the too high amount of sugar. In Europe, approximately 53 million inhabitants are affected either by Type 1 Diabetes Mellitus or Type 2 Diabetes Mellitus (ÖDG, N.D.).

In Austria, it is estimated that about 600.000 people are suffering from Diabetes while approximately 20% of the affected persons are unaware of their disease. Diabetes Mellitus can lead to serious second diseases like heart attack, stroke, amputations, etc. which is the reason, why corrective measures have to be implemented in order to decrease the prevalence of Diabetes. Risk factors are similar to the ones of the other non-communicable diseases – people who are less educated, have less income or do have a migration background are more often affected by obesity and are therefore at higher risk to develop Diabetes. (BMGF, 2017)

2.2 HEALTH PROMOTION AND PREVENTION PROGRAMS

Health promotion and prevention are two processes, that might seem similar to each other but differ slightly in both their execution and definition. First of all, an understanding of the definition of "health" is needed. The WHO described health in their constitution as "*a state of complete physical, mental and social well-being and not merely the absence of disease or infirmity. The enjoyment of the highest attainable standard of health is one of the fundamental rights of every human being without distinction of race, religion, political belief, economic or social condition.*" (WHO, 2018). Therefore, being healthy signifies more than just feeling physically well.

But what can we do to achieve and maintain a healthy life? Health promotion is based on the knowledge about which factors increase the chance for a healthy life (the chance for an increased amount of healthy life years) and aims at promoting these factors (Fonds Gesundes Österreich, N.D.). Health promotion programs are therefore <u>unspecific measures</u> that aim at an increased population health – e.g. a hiking day within the company, physical exercise at work, etc.

Prevention, on the opposite, is based on the knowledge about what weakens and harms the health state and strives after reducing those factors (Fond Gesundes Österreich, N.D.). In detail, prevention programs are <u>specific measures</u> to increase the population health. Prevention programs can furthermore be divided into three parts, which differ from each other in their definition:

Primary Prevention = activities to reduce the incidence of the disease and the individual risk of the disease <u>before damage is observable</u>.

Secondary Prevention = activities to <u>early detect</u> a disease in order to reduce the morbidity and to increase the chance of survival at the same time (e.g. screening).

Tertiary Prevention = activities to <u>reduce social and medical consequences</u> of an established disease (e.g. rehabilitation).

Besides the different segmentations of prevention measures there are also different prevention strategies, from which I want to outline two.

2.2.1 The High-Risk Approach

The high-risk approach (*see: Figure 2*) describes clinical, individual prevention. Its practices are <u>counselling</u> to change the individual risk behaviour, <u>medication</u> to delay the occurrence of the disease and <u>screening</u> to early detect an asymptomatic disease. Examples for a high-risk approach are: breast cancer screening, blood pressure checks, safe sex counselling, etc. Basically, the high-risk strategy can also be compared to a "face to face intervention", as it controls the individual behaviour.

The positive aspects about this strategy are, that the intervention is appropriate for an individual at risk and that there is a favourable benefit-risk ratio. Furthermore, the motivation for an intervention like this is high for both, the physician and the subject (= individual).

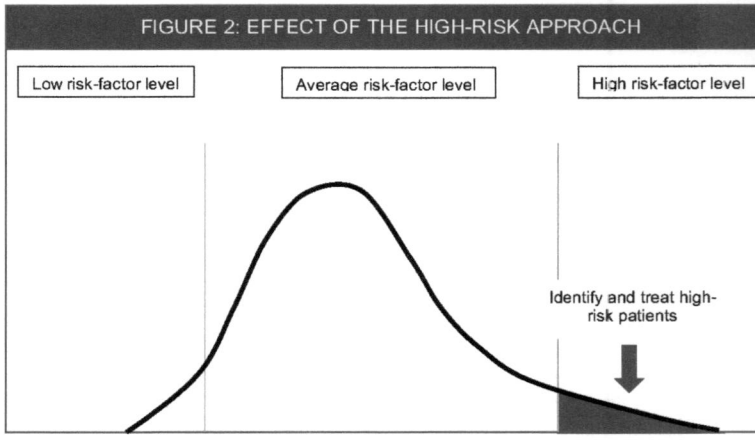

FIGURE 2: EFFECT OF THE HIGH-RISK APPROACH

Low risk-factor level Average risk-factor level High risk-factor level

Identify and treat high-risk patients

Negatives, that should be outlined are, that the costs for high-risk interventions are extremely high most of the time (e.g. screening). Secondly, the potential for the whole population is limited.

2.2.2 The Population Approach

The population approach (*see: Figure 3*) is, as the name already says, a population based intervention. It aims at modifying community determinants. Examples are: water supply protection, a smoke free environment or nutritional programs to name a few. The population strategy is also known as the "mass approach" as its target is to control the determinants of risk factors for the whole population.

The positive aspect about this strategy is, that the impact for the population as a whole is high even though there is only a small benefit for the participating individuals as such. This situation leads up to the so called "prevention paradox" which describes the fact, that a preventive measure brings much benefit to the population but offers little to each individual.

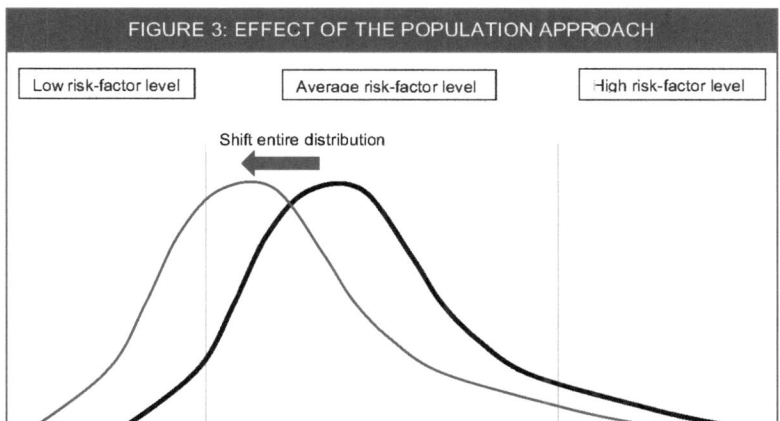

FIGURE 3: EFFECT OF THE POPULATION APPROACH

Low risk-factor level | Average risk-factor level | High risk-factor level

Shift entire distribution

On the other hand, the benefit-risk ratio of these interventions is worrisome. Even though the costs depend on the specific measure, the motivation for both the physician and the individual is rather low.

There are several examples, how health promotion and prevention programs can be implemented – one specific, also concerning the technical advantages nowadays, will be explained now.

"Sidekickhealth" is an evidence-based mobile platform to prevent and treat lifestyle related non-communicable diseases. The project is basically a social-health game and service for smartphones that allows people to improve their health and well-being by doing different activities in three categories. Those categories are: food (nutrition), mind (mental health) and exercise (physical health). "Sidekickhealth" can be used by providers or employers within a company and is "*a unique combination of behavioural economics, the latest in gaming technology and artificial intelligence*" (Sidekickhealth, 2018). This invention shows, that digitalization and the technical progress can be combined with interventions that aim at a better health state of a certain group of people. To some extent, this service even uses artificial intelligence, even only at a very small scale, as everyone who uses this service, starts with different preconditions – but everyone will get the same "reward" after finishing a certain goal. Therefore, the app adapts very fast to the individual and supports him or her with a fitness or diet plan, fitting the respective needs and tracking their activities.

However, before trying to link artificial intelligence with its possibilities in the healthcare sector, the term itself has to be defined.

3. ARTIFICIAL INTELLIGENCE

Digitalisation and its effects, new inventions and methods are not anymore just a rare phenomenon – the process of rapid modernization became reality over the past years. Communication, marketing, consuming, just to name a few processes – everything gets done by online tools following certain algorithms in order to produce the outcome we expect. Most people do not even recognize, that they are using artificial intelligence and machine learning in their everyday routine. Navigation apps, streaming services, intelligent home personal assistants or smart home assistants – all of those services feature elements of artificial intelligence. To support this argument, a research on how many US citizens are already using machine learning services to some extent was done and published by the Gallup Incorporation. The outcome was, that nearly nine out of ten Americans stated, that they use "*at least one of six devices, programs or services that feature elements of artificial intelligence (AI)*" (Gallup, 2018).

The definition of artificial intelligence, nevertheless, includes more than just knowing what song title we want to listen to next. Artificial intelligence is defined as "*an area of computer science that emphasizes the creation of intelligent machines and reacts like humans. (…) Knowledge engineering is a core part of AI research*" (Techopedia, 2019). Artificial intelligence is therefore used to describe the process, when a machine (or more specific: a software) is gaining knowledge on its own, analysing and evaluating the gathered data and to improve its performance on the specific task based on the retrieved information. A robot, for example, featuring artificial intelligence elements can act like a human being, in most cases even more precise, faster and way more efficient.

3.1 HISTORICAL DEVELOPMENT

In the following paragraphs, significant milestones for the development of artificial intelligence and machine learning will be listed and explained briefly in order to both get a rough overview on how this specific field changed but also gained interest and attention over time and to gather a more detailed understanding on what AI is about.

The historical development of artificial intelligence as we know it today, had its beginning a long time ago. The idea of a logical argument, or even the succession of more logical arguments, that come to a certain conclusion based on a number of conditionals, has already emerged around 350 BC, when the Greek philosopher Aristotle came up with the idea of the so-called *syllogism* (Smiley, 1973). As Aristotle lived from 384 BC until 322 BC, his ideas did not really have an impact on artificial intelligence, even though the basic assumption was more or less the same.

Nevertheless, in 1950, the famous "Computing Machinery and Intelligence" article by Alan Turing was published in the journal *Mind* (Moor, 2003). In this article, the popular *Turing-Test* was described. The test was basically about three parties: A – a human being, B – a computer and C – an interrogator, again a human being. The aim was, to test the machine's (B) ability, to what extent it can mimic human behaviour to a variety of questions. While all parties where separated from each other, C had to find out, based on the answers the other two parties gave on specific questions, which answers are computer-generated and which answers were given by the real person. As this test specifically analysed the machine-learning-process, or much more the ability of a computer to exhibit intelligent behaviour equivalent to human behaviour, it is often called the first milestone in the history of artificial intelligence. (Turing, 1950)

13 years later, in 1963, a collection of articles referring to artificial intelligence called *Computers and Thought* was published by Edward Feigenbaum, computer scientist, and Julian Feldman. The reports analysed in the book are "*concerned with the information processing activity that underlies intelligent behaviour in human beings and computers*" (Feigenbaum & Feldman, 1963). Feigenbaum, nevertheless, developed a software using machine learning two years after his publication: Dendral, the first expert system. Feigenbaum therefore set the beginning of a software operated computer, that is able to retrieve expert's data out of huge databases and then finish the process of decision-making off based on logical arguments – Dendral was basically written "to solve problems of inductive inference in organic chemistry" (Buchanan, Feigenbaum & Lederberg, 1970).

> **Expert system** = software, that makes use of "expert knowledge" in order to come up with an advice on how to solve a specific problem. Those systems are "*particularly useful and necessary when the decision situation is not adequately structured to use decision support systems. They are being aimed at (…) situations in which an expert's knowledge is needed to find at least acceptable solutions*" (Zimmermann, 2012).

In the 2000s, artificial intelligence experienced a tremendous increase in both public interest but also in software inventions using machine learning. Not only did interactive computers and robots become commercially available but also organizations like the NASA implemented AI into their existing processes. AI then became available to the vast majority in the 2010s when Apple introduced its voice assistant *Siri*, Google combined its navigation services with AI and Microsoft launched an additional gaming device for its console – *Kinect* -, that was able to track human body movements, enabling people to play videogames just by moving their body.

The status quo regarding artificial intelligence for consumers reached a point where people do not even have to call their hairdresser or at a restaurant for example anymore in order to fix an appointment – smart assistants, like *Google Duplex*, will have a phone call for you, they will have a natural conversation with the other party (Leviathan, 2018). To put that in other words, computers can have real conversations with real people, respond to their answers and learn throughout the conversation. But not only for consumers AI became interesting, also for businesses – logistics, for example, can be fully done by a software featuring machine learning skills. Those kinds of software are usually way more precise, efficient and, nevertheless, cheaper in total than a human resource.

4. ARTIFICIAL INTELLIGENCE IN THE HEALTHCARE SECTOR

The following section will act as a conclusion of this literature review – both benefits but also risks when implementing software based on machine learning will be stressed and discussed. Therefore, the listing of those aspects summarizes the discussion on the use of AI in healthcare.

4.1 BENEFITS

Implementing artificial intelligence in different processes in the healthcare system would come with a variety of benefits, not only for the patients but also for the system as such, regarding savings of billions of Euros.

Firstly, the PwC study "Sherlock in Health" (PwC, 2017) showed, that the implementation of artificial intelligence promises a significant development in early detecting grave diseases like dementia or breast cancer. Regarding dementia, it will be possible to combine old and new procedures – the diagnosis therefore will be possible even before the affected persons notice a change in their cognitive behaviour. A clinical study from the Netherlands stated, that AI-methods can be combined with conventional diagnosis methods like the magnetic resonance imaging system (MRI system) in order to detect Alzheimer's in an early stadium with an accuracy of nearly 90% (Med Device Online, 2016). Concerning the benefit in the diagnosis of breast cancer, the study found, that nearly 30% of all cancer incidents are categorised as breast cancer. At the moment of the study in 2017, the incidence in Austria was stated with 90,7, meaning that per year 91 women are diagnosed with this disease. Artificial intelligence will help analysing the mammography-results 30 times faster than by a doctor with an error rate of only one percent. Furthermore, AI will also be able to tell how a person will react to different kinds of chemotherapies – this will again lead to a speculated saving of €74 billion in the next ten years.

Secondly, Austria can be found in the EU-wide top places regarding the spending on healthcare – Austria spent €33,8 billion, which is equivalent to 19,3% of the GDP) on its healthcare system in 2014. This amount of money is likely to increase tremendously as the population as a whole becomes older (it is expected, that by 2014 26% of Europe's population will be older than 65). Therefore, implementing artificial intelligence will be a crucial part for the declared long-term goal to use resources more efficiently – meaning: to spend less by acquiring a higher and better outcome for everyone. Not only the analysing and diagnosing process will be faster and cheaper, also operations can be automatized. (PwC, 2017)

However, AI and the early diagnoses as a consequence of its implementation will also lead to better and more efficient therapies. With the use of AI software, it will be possible to already detect obesity, or at least detect the risk of being affected by obesity, in the database of a two-year old. As a consequence, doctors but also parents are given the possibility to react a lot earlier to the disease. Nevertheless, another benefit in this clinical picture is, that hopefully in a few years it will be possible to state, if the respective obesity is caused by the personal lifestyle, the eating/diet habits or by the genetic preposition which will automatically also lead to better therapy possibilities. (PwC, 2017)

4.2 RISKS

Nevertheless, besides all the positive aspects, also the risks, AI comes along with, need to be focussed on.

First of all, it will take some time to set up the framework conditions for a successful implementation of artificial intelligence in the healthcare sector. That means, that AI works on huge databases and datasets that need to be set up properly before it can be worked with them. The setting up process comes along with a certain amount of risk as a lack of data, or even the existence of wrong data, will lead to discrimination. (PwC, 2017). This would result in grave problems, as it will be hard to exactly to find out where the initial lack of information was.

Furthermore, new risks arising from the field of cyber criminality need to be taken into consideration (Salzburger Nachrichten, 2018). Personal data and personal privacy might be exposed to a high risk of not being private anymore. It is therefore necessary, to concern human rights when implementing AI software whilst ensuring a high level of security of data. But cyber criminality is not only affecting personal privacy – artificial intelligence might also be a risk to future democratic decisions due to the spread of information generated by a software, not by humans anymore.

However, there are already plans for Austria on how to face those challenges. The whitepaper of the Austrian council for robotics and artificial intelligence (Österreichischer Rat für Robotik und Künstliche Intelligenz, 2018) revealed a clear strategy, how Austria will implement AI step by step in different fields. In this paper, it is also stated, that the council wants to implement measures in order to early detect potential sources of risk for society. Also, a legal framework should be established with the aim to secure the safety of AI. Raising awareness among the population, however, is also on the priority list, meaning that educational trainings on this topic should be stressed while AI should also be implemented in the field of the police.

BIBLIOGRAPHY

Amt der Tiroler Landesregierung. (2013). *Tiroler Gesundheitsbericht 2012*. Amt der Tiroler Landesregierung. Retrieved from: https://www.tirol.gv.at/fileadmin/themen/ gesundheitvorsorge/influenza/downloads/TLGB2012.pdf on February 25th, 2019.

BMGF. (2017). *Österreichische Diabetes-Strategie*. Bundesministerium für Gesundheit & Frauen Österreich GmbH, Wien. Retrieved from: https://www.bmgf.gv.at/cms/home/attachments/2/7/2/CH1075/CMS1460386129805/diabetes strategie.pdf on February 27th, 2019.

Buchanan, B., Feigenbaum, E. & Lederberg, J. (1970). *On Generality and Problem Solving: A Case Study using the Dendral Program*. Computer Science Department Stanford University. Retrieved from: https://ntrs.nasa.gov/archive/nasa/casi.ntrs.nasa.gov/19710028679.pdf on February 27th, 2019.

Engelgau, M., Rosenhouse, S., et al. (2011). *The Economic Effect of Noncommunicable Diseases on Households and Nations: A Review of Existing Evidence* published in: Journal of Health Communication Vol. 16 in 2011. Retrieved from: http://www.tandfonline.com/doi/abs/10.1080/10810730.2011.601394 on February 25th, 2019.

Feigenbaum, E. & Feldman, J. (1963). *Computers and Thought*. McGraw-Hill Book Company. Retrieved from: https://stacks.stanford.edu/file/druid:mb725bt3951/mb725bt3951.pdf on February 27th, 2019.

Fonds Gesundes Österreich. (N.D.). *1x1 der Gesundheitsförderung*. Retrieved from: http://fgoe.org/1x1_der_Gesundheitsfoerderung on February 25th, 2019.

Gallup Inc. (2018). *Most Americans Already Using Artificial Intelligence Products*. Retrieved from: https://news.gallup.com/poll/228497/americans-already-using-artificial-intelligence-products.aspx on February 26th, 2019.

Griebler, R., Anzenberger, J., & Eisenmann, A. (2014). *Herz-Kreislauf-Erkrankungen in Österreich: Angina Pectoris, Myokardinfarkt, ischämischer Schlaganfall, periphere arterielle Verschlusskrankheit. Epidemiologie und Prävention*. Wien, Bundesministerium für Gesundheit

International Agency for Research on Cancer. (2014). *World Cancer Report 2014*. Distributed by WHO Press

Leviathan, Y. (2018). *Google Duplex: An AI System for Accomplishing Real-World Tasks over the Phone*. Posted on: Google AI Blog. Retrieved from: https://ai.googleblog.com/2018/05/duplex-ai-system-for-natural-conversation.html on February 27th, 2019.

Med Device Online. (2016). *Artificial Intelligence Could Aid Earlier Diagnosis of Alzheimer's*. Retrieved from: https://www.meddeviceonline.com/doc/artificial-intelligence-could-aid-earlier-diagnosis-of-alzheimer-s-0001 on February 26th, 2019.

Moor, J. (2003). *The Turing Test: The Elusive Standard of Artificial Intelligence*. Springer Science & Business Media.

Neue Züricher Zeitung. (2015). *Nur einer von zwanzig Menschen weltweit ist gesund*. Retrieved from: https://www.nzz.ch/wissenschaft/medizin/nur-einer-von-zwanzig-menschen-weltweit-ist-gesund-1.18558064 on February 25th, 2019.

ÖDG. (N.D.). *31. Österreichischer Diabetestag*. Österreichische Diabetes Gesellschaft. Retrieved from: http://www.oedg.at/patienten/1710-31-oesterreichische-diabetestag on February 26th, 2019.

Österreichischer Rat für Robotik und Künstliche Intelligenz. (2018). *Die Zukunft Österreichs mit Robotik und Künstlicher Intelligenz positiv gestalten – White Paper des Österreichischen Rats für Robotik und Künstliche Intelligenz*. Retrieved from: https://www.acrai.at/images/download/ACRAI_whitebook_online_2018.pdf on February 25th, 2019.

PwC. (2017). *Sherlock in Health – How artificial intelligence may improve quality and efficienty whilst reducing healthcare costs in Europe*. Retrieved from: https://www.pwc.at/de/publikationen/branchen-und-wirtschaftsstudien/pwc_sherlock_in_health_0717.pdf on February 26th,2019.

Salzburger Nachrichten. (2018). *Österreich bekommt Strategie für Künstliche Intelligenz*. Retrieved from: https://www.sn.at/panorama/oesterreich/oesterreich-bekommt-strategie-fuer-kuenstliche-intelligenz-61476547 on February 26th, 2019.

Sidekickhealth. (2018). *Sidekickhealth – Improve your Health the Fun Way*. Retrieved from: https://sidekickhealth.com/ on February 26th,2019.

Silverstein, A., Silverstein, L., & Silverstein, V. (2006). *Cancer: Conquering a Deadly Disease*. Twenty-First Century Books

Smiley, T.J. (1973). *What is a syllogism?* in: Journal of Philosophic Logic, January 1973, Volume 2, pp 136. Retrieved from: https://link.springer.com/article/10.1007%2FBF02115614?LI=true on February 26th, 2019.

Techopedia Inc. (2019). *Artificial Intelligence (AI) – Definition: What does Artificial Intelligence (AI) mean?* Retrieved from: https://www.techopedia.com/definition/190/artificial-intelligence-ai on February 26th, 2019.

Turing, A.M. (1950). *Computing Machinery and Intelligence* in: MIND Volume 59, No. 236, pp 433 – 460. Retrieved from: https://bit.ly/2IUaCQX on February 26th 2019.
WHO. (2014). *Noncommunicable Diseases – Country Profiles 2014*. World Health Organisation. Retrieved from: http://apps.who.int/iris/bitstream/10665/128038/1/9789241507509_eng.pdf on February 26th, 2019.

WHO. (2014). *Noncommunicable Diseases – Country Profiles 2014*. World Health Organisation. Retrieved from: http://apps.who.int/iris/bitstream/10635/128038/1/9789241507509_eng.pdf on February 26th, 2019.

WHO. (2017). *Noncommunicable diseases – factsheet*. World Health Organisation. Retrieved from: : http://www.who.int/mediacentre/factsheets/fs355/en/ on February 25th, 2019.

WHO. (2018). *Constitution of the World Health Organization*. World Health Organisation. Retrieved from: http://apps.who.int/gb/bd/PDF/bd47/EN/constitution-en.pdf?ua=1 on February 25th, 2019.

WHO Regional Office for Europe. (N.D.). *Health systems response to NCD's*. World Health Organisation. Retrieved from: http://www.euro.who.int/en/health-topics/Health-systems/health-systems-response-to-ncds/health-systems-response-to-ncds on February 25th, 2019.

Zimmermann, H.J. (2012). *Fuzzy Sets, Decision Making, and Expert Systems*. Springer Science & Business Media. Retrieved from: https://books.google.at/books?hl=de&lr=&id=-PfnCAAAQBAJ&oi=fnd&pg=PA1&dq=expert+system+definition&ots=3JJya9dFDR&sig=Sq0H0R7oHxatenVMpJnzlyww-j0#v=onepage&q=expert%20system%20definition&f=false on February 27th, 2019.

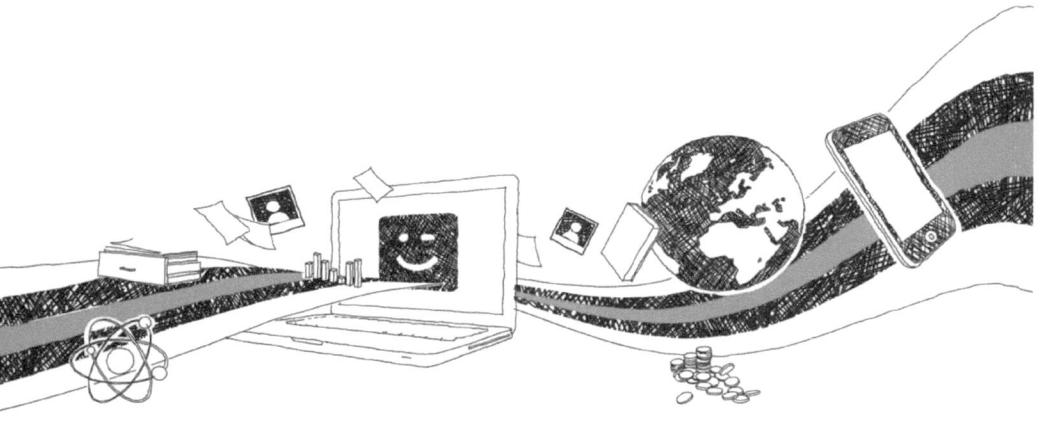
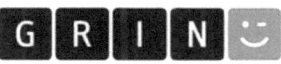